Down Syndrome and Dementia

SHARING GOOD PRACTICE SERIES

Down Syndrome and Dementia

A Guide for Family Members, Social and
Health Care Staff and Students

Bob Dawson RMN, RNLD

THE CHOIR PRESS

First published in the United Kingdom in 2020 by
The Choir Press

ISBN 978-1-78963-167-8

Acknowledgements

Many thanks to Dee, who not only tolerated me when writing but also actively supported by proof reading and adding many valuable suggestions to the text.

Many thanks to Tracy for proof reading as a recently retired care manager and for her valuable suggestions.

Also, many thanks to Marg, Catherine and Jed for proof reading using their family experiences.

I would like to thank my editor Josh, together with colleagues Rachel, Adrian and Miles at The Choir Press for their combined help and support to turn my manuscript into a finished book.

Contents

Introduction

Hello, my name is Bob Dawson. My background has always been in health and social care. I qualified in mental health and learning disability nursing during the 1980s working up to the level of nursing officer within the Health Service, then moved as a senior manager into social care within the voluntary/charitable sector in 1991. Since then I have been involved in education and development, consultancy and training, which became my full-time job from 1999.

My experiences supporting people with Down syndrome and dementia and their families include managing a specific Down syndrome and dementia service from 1991–1995 with the Hansel Alliance, a learning disability charity based in Symington Ayrshire. During this time, I was involved with an international working group, researching the prevalence of dementia within the Down syndrome population, per age groups, and common symptoms they experienced.

At this time, I was also Ayrshire and Arran Health Board's representative on an international working group, chaired by Emeritus Professor Tony Holland CBE, Cambridge University, whose aims were to pool, share and develop this relatively new area of research.

Currently I develop training and development packages for carers and families and provide consultancy for teams supporting people with Down syndrome and dementia.

Organisations I have worked with include South Gloucestershire, North Somerset and Bath and North East Somerset Councils, Hansel Alliance, Scottish and English Down Syndrome Associations, Milestones Trust, Care, Camphill Communities, Visions, Home Farm Trust, ARC, Scope, Lodge Trust, Stirling University Dementia Resources Unit, Dementia Voice and many others.

Over the last decade, when training in this area, the format has been quite simple. I ask participants to raise their questions about dementia and how the individuals they support are affected by their dementia.

Participants raise their questions on flip-chart paper, and we spend the rest of the training day answering their questions. I have found, and participants have agreed, that this is the most effective way of addressing the needs of all participants, as well as covering all the areas that are important for carers to know.

This publication aims to replicate the training and development session using the questions asked over the years to form an index.

There is no need to read the book systematically front to back; you can choose to go to the questions you want to know the answers to first.

This is not an academic publication (see the appendix at the end of this book for useful websites for those who want to read more). It is aimed at family members, support workers, students and others supporting individuals with Down syndrome and dementia. Some of the information is anecdotal, coming from over 40 years of experience in working in the area and from the many people I have trained during this time.

Over the years I have met many hundreds of people with Down syndrome who had dementia. They were all individuals, with very individual needs.

It is important not to define a person based on their diagnosis alone. My firm, long-held belief is that when trying to meet people's needs, if you plan their support based only on their diagnosis, you have already failed to recognise their uniqueness.

Person-centred care and support means not only meeting the day-to-day needs of an individual but also ensuring that we are first recognising the person's personality, their life experiences, opportunities, upbringing and personal wishes and beliefs. You need to establish the impact of the diagnosis on the person and then negotiate and plan support appropriately, involving the person as much as they are able.

Before you start looking for the answers to your questions, I think it is important to note: research in this area is ongoing and some aspects of current thinking may well change as we learn more.

To keep you up to date with further research I request you only read information from reputable resources who check the authenticity of information they put on their various websites. A list of these organisations in the UK are included in the appendix at the end of this book.

Every question you have ever had, answered

1. What is Down syndrome?

Down syndrome is a chromosomal condition where the individual has a third copy of all or part of chromosome 21. It is the most common cause of intellectual impairment and learning difficulty. Around 1 in every 1,000 births a year in the UK will have Down syndrome. There are 40,000–60,000 people in the UK with the condition. Today the average life expectancy for a person with Down syndrome is between 50–60. In 1983 the average lifespan of a person with Down syndrome was 25 years. (See answer to Question 4 for more details).

The condition was named after Dr Langdon Down, who in 1862 first described this genetic condition. As Dr Langdon Down did not have Down syndrome himself the correct terminology is Down syndrome, not Down's Syndrome. (My thanks to Blanche Nicolson MBE who set me straight on this issue back in 1991.)

2. Are there different types of Down syndrome?

Yes. There are three types:

Trisomy 21 (92–95% of cases): Each cell in the body has 23 pairs of chromosomes, 46 in total. In Trisomy 21 there is a complete extra copy of chromosome 21 meaning 47 chromosomes in total.

Translocation (2.5%): The long arm of chromosome 21 is attached to another chromosome, usually chromosome 14.

Mosaic (1–2.5%): Some cells are normal, having 46 chromosomes, and others have the extra chromosome 21.

3. What are the characteristics of Down syndrome?

It is important to look at the characteristics of Down syndrome because some of these inherent issues are relevant if they develop dementia and can be planned for to minimise potential future problems.

Some or all the following characteristics will be present in people who have Down syndrome:

- Flat back of the head.
- Abundant neck skin.
- Fat facial appearance.
- Slanted eyes.
- Epicanthic folds – this is a skin fold of the upper eyelid covering the inner corner of the eye.
- Speckling of the iris – Brushfield's spots.
- Small teeth.
- Furrowed tongue – these last two can lead to problems when dementia occurs, such as swallowing and choking issues.
- Short, broad hands.
- Bent fifth fingertip.
- Single transverse palmar crease – a single line that runs across the palm of the hand (people most often have three creases in their palms), affecting approximately 1 in 30 in the general population.
- A wide space between the first and second toes.
- Gastrointestinal abnormalities – the most common being reflux, obesity, constipation and diarrhoea. About 5% will develop celiac disease.
- Congenital heart defects – this can lead to problems when dementia occurs, see answer to Question 5.
- Muscle hypotonia – low muscle tone.

- Hyper-extensibility or hyper-flexibility – ligaments and joints are much more flexible.
- Cervical spine instability.
- Shortness of stature, at the bottom end of the range.

4. Why are people with Down syndrome now living longer?

While there are many reasons the life expectancy of people with Down syndrome has increased dramatically, I will list the four main ones.

- **The use of antibiotics.** It is important to remember that antibiotics were first used towards the end of the Second World War, the mid-1940s. Coupled with an increased susceptibility to infections, this left the person with Down syndrome more at risk before this time.
- **The development of immunisation programmes** in the 1960s, i.e. measles, 1963; mumps, 1967; and rubella, 1969. These were combined into the MMR vaccine in 1971. Prior to this substantial numbers of people died of these diseases each year. With large communal living conditions and susceptibility to infection this left the Down syndrome group more at risk.
- **The development and use of heart surgery** to correct congenital heart defects that affect 40–50% of people with Down syndrome. While younger people have benefited from these improvements there is still a major issue with, primarily, the over 50s for whom the surgery was not available.
- **The move away from institutional care** and the development of community care provision both in people's own homes and supported accommodation. This has helped increase life expectancy for people with Down syndrome, because:

- Living conditions are much more favourable. In the institutions ward sizes were large with, often, 45+ people sharing the same space. When you have a group who are more susceptible to infections, the individuals with Down syndrome are often disproportionally affected. Nowadays people with learning difficulties predominantly live in community settings where numbers are much smaller and therefore safer.
- Many people with Down syndrome are sociable and amenable and have integrated well into local communities and been accepted as members of those communities. This has in turn created a more purposeful, stimulating, and meaningful life for this group. Therefore, there is much less chronic boredom and frustration that was present within the more restrictive environment of institutional living.

5. What are common health issues for the person with Down syndrome?

- Hypothyroidism – the area where I have most often come across individuals with a misdiagnosis, as the symptoms of hypothyroidism and dementia are similar. This is less a problem now than it was 20 years ago. It should be automatic now that part of the diagnostic process requires blood tests looking for metabolic disorders such as thyroid problems and diabetes.
- Eye problems including cataracts, strabismus (squint) and refractive errors such as near-sightedness, far-sightedness and blurred vision.
- Spine disturbance atlantoaxial instability affecting the top two vertebrae of the neck.
- Susceptibility to infections due to a poor immune system.

Therefore, infections like respiratory, urinary, skin, and those spread by contact with others are more common in this group.

- Sleep disturbance – sleep apnoea, where, during sleep, a person will suddenly stop breathing and then start again.
- Congenital heart abnormalities affect 40–50% of people who have Down syndrome – for example, atrial septal defect, atrioventricular septal defect and AVSD with Fallot's. (Much more information is available on https://dhg.org.uk/information/)

  This is an area of concern for people with Down syndrome who develop dementia.

  I have known of a significant number of people who have died because of heart failure early in their dementia diagnosis. One of the effects of dementia is a reduction in white blood cells, needed to fight infection. As people who have Down syndrome are generally more susceptible to infection, this added risk can place greater pressure on the heart.
- Hearing – primarily glue ear and nerve deafness.
- Obesity.
- Gastrointestinal defects – which may include abnormalities of the intestines, oesophagus and trachea.

6. Why are so many people with Down syndrome overweight?

The medical reason for this is that many people with Down syndrome have hypothyroidism and therefore a lower metabolic rate. This results in them being more prone to weight gain.

In addition, however, there have been social reasons which have historically influenced weight gain. We, in the care and support field, need to recognise how our behaviours can affect the health of the people we support in both a positive and, as in this case, a negative way.

If you are working with someone who is sociable and amenable, who regularly smiles and engages with you, as is the case for many people who have Down syndrome, then you are more psychologically predisposed to give them more treats and outings. In addition, life in the institutions was generally more sedentary: therefore, lack of exercise was also a contributing factor.

In the next 20 years it will be interesting to see if we look back on obesity within the Down syndrome group as another problem greatly eased by the closure of the institutions with people now living more active lives with increased purpose.

7. What is dementia?

The term dementia is the umbrella term used to describe the progressive symptoms that occur when the brain is affected by specific diseases and conditions. According to the World Health Organisation (September 2019) dementia is typified by: deterioration of memory, thinking, behaviour and the ability to perform everyday activities.

Each person is unique and will experience dementia in their own way, however, symptoms usually include loss of memory, difficulties with problem solving, mood changes and communication problems.

8. Is Alzheimer's the same as dementia, or are there different types?

According to Dementia UK there are over 200 subtypes of dementia. Let's break this down into manageable chunks.

- The largest single group are people with **Alzheimer's Disease.** This group accounts for most people with Down syndrome who develop dementia. First recorded by Dr Alois Alzheimer, a German psychiatrist, in the early 1900s, it is typified by a loss of brain cells on the surface and deep within the brain, as well as a gradual decline of functions over a lengthy period. If you speak to family or staff at six-month intervals, they often describe little change; this is partly because the process is slow and partly because they are subconsciously adapting to the changes in the individual as they happen.
- **Lewy body dementia.** This was first described by Dr Fredrich H. Lewy in the early 1900s, typified by symptoms including hallucinations, delusions, mobility problems similar to Parkinson, agnosia (misinterpreting sensory stimulation), altered visual perception (e.g. floral carpets can appear to be 3D), proneness to falls and sleep disturbance.
- **Vascular dementia.** This form of dementia is caused by reduced blood flow to the brain, which occurs where there is a narrowing and blockage of the small blood vessels inside the brain. This can happen after a single stroke where the blood supply to an area of the brain is cut off, or more commonly where the individual has many 'small strokes' (transient ischemic attacks) that may cause small but widespread damage to the brain.
- The majority of diagnosed dementias fall into the above three types. However, they can also be caused by any of the following:

- Toxic substances such as lead, cadmium, mercury and alcohol, e.g. Korsakoff syndrome.
- Infective diseases affecting the brain, e.g. neuro-syphilis, Creutzfeldt-Jakob disease.
- Degenerative disease processes that affect the brain such as Pick's disease, Huntington's disease, Parkinson disease.
- Head injury, e.g. road traffic accident, falling from a height, assault, boxing.
- It is also not uncommon for the individual to have more than one type of dementia, or to have no known cause.

9. Is dementia on the increase?

This is one of the most frequently asked questions.

In the general population there are two main reasons for the current reported increase in the number of people being diagnosed as having dementia.

The first reason for this is that, as a result of the National Health Service being founded in 1948, providing free health care, including maternity services, for all following the end of the Second World War, there was a baby boom. This ended in 1961 when contraception became available on the NHS.

Approximately twice as many babies were born and survived during these years compared to the period before WW2.

People born during that period are now aged between 59 and 72 years. Therefore, most of the current increase is not due to an underlying increase in dementia but more that there are more people in the age group who are more vulnerable to developing dementia.

Secondly, again predominantly as a result of the creation of the NHS and improved general health and improvement in treatments and cures for previously life-limiting conditions, average life expectancy has increased dramatically, approximately 60 yrs in 1930s to 80 yrs+ today.

In the Down syndrome population, it is almost entirely due to increased life expectancy for the reasons explained in Question 4.

The first recorded cases of Down syndrome and dementia were by Fraser & Mitchell, 1876, who stated that 'death was attributed to nothing more than general decay, a sort of precipitated senility' (*an early term for dementia*). Most of our current knowledge stems from research started in the 1980s which continues today as greater numbers of people are living to an age when dementia was and continues to be more prevalent.

10. How common is dementia in Down syndrome?

It is useful to look at the rates of dementia in the general population and compare this with dementia in Down syndrome.

Currently in the UK approximately 7–10% of over-65s will develop dementia, rising to 20–24% for the over-80s.

In Down syndrome the percentages are much higher. Between 40–49 years around 8%, between 50–59 years around 55% and over-60 years around 75%. Some sources quote slightly different figures. However, the research I have carried out within the Hansel Alliance (Ayrshire, Scotland) in 1994 and within the Phoenix Trust in 1998 (Bristol, now closed) matched the above statistics.

Around 98% of diagnosed cases had Alzheimer's disease and in 2% the cause was vascular.

11. Why is the percentage much higher in people with Down syndrome?

Most individuals with Down syndrome have deposits of beta-amyloid plaques and tau tangles laid down in the brain by the age of 40. In the general population these are evidence of Alzheimer's disease.

However, it is important to note that despite having these deposits, over 25% of people who have Down syndrome do not develop dementia. The reason for this is not currently known.

Scientists believe that dementia, as with other health issues for individuals with Down syndrome, are as a result of the extra chromosome 21. This is an area of active research and, in the future, we are hopeful there will be more accurate and useful information.

12. What are the early warning signs of dementia in this group?

Both this question and Question 21 are taken from research I carried out at Hansel Alliance in Symington Ayrshire.

Here I worked with many individuals with Down syndrome. The organisation also, at that time, had a ten-bedded home dedicated to meet the needs of people with dementia.

This research at the Hansel Alliance was published in a book by Diana Kerr: *Down Syndrome and Dementia* in 1997, by Venture Press.

I was also actively involved with Scope in Ayr, which increased the number of Down syndrome individuals I had regular contact with.

Since this time, I have continued researching commonly seen symptoms, through my role as a consultant and trainer in various locations in the UK but primarily in the South West of England.

The following are thirteen common symptoms described by family members or carers concerned about changes in the individual with Down syndrome that invariably lead to a diagnosis of dementia.

- **Seizures.** Around 60% will develop epileptic activity in the early stage. To date every person with Down syndrome that I have known who has developed seizures, having had no previous history of epilepsy, has later been diagnosed with dementia.

    I have, on the other hand, met individuals with Down syndrome and long-term epilepsy who have not developed dementia.
- **Apathy and general inactivity.** This must be measured against the normal mood and activity of the individual.
- **Short-term memory loss.** This can be very difficult to assess, dependent on the level of the person's learning disability, because for many we act as their memory, reminding individuals about routine, appointments and all aspects of their life. We need to quantify on an individual basis what memory means for the individual so we can detect changes. (See also Question 17.)
- **Loss of daily living skills.** Again, this is dependent on changes from the norm for the individual and could range from dressing to cooking, from reading to going out to the shops.
- **Loss of amenability and sociability.** Can I set the record straight: not all individuals with Down syndrome are amenable and sociable, however, many are. In this group you can expect changes caused by the effects of dementia. The changes may include previously unseen, increased levels of frustration, swearing and preoccupation.
- **Loss of interest** in favoured hobbies and activities. For some this may be no longer watching a favourite programme on TV, for others it could be not wanting to go to a favoured club or losing interest in activities such as reading, painting or gardening.

- **Withdrawal of spontaneous communication.** You know the individuals you support. You know their normal communication. When you enter their space, someone may have a common greeting for you. They may have a unique way of showing happiness or sadness. With the onset of dementia these unique communications are likely to diminish.
- **Loss of road sense.** It is important that when you are concerned an individual may be developing dementia that you reassess their road skills. Note in the general population this skill can remain for a much longer time than in people with learning difficulties.
- **Disorientation and confusion,** when compared to what is normal for the individual.
- **Loss of comprehension.** Not appearing to comprehend what was previously understood in conversations, requests, instructions. Not easily becoming involved in discussions that previously they would have had an opinion or comment on.
- **Increased purposeful walking.** This was previously described as 'wandering' but this implies that there is no purpose to the walking. But that is not an accurate description as most people with dementia walk with a purpose; our job is to work out, if possible, what that purpose is. (See also answer to Questions 29 and 30).
- **Visual spatial problems.** Misinterpreting shadows, stepping over lines in the carpet.
- **Depression.** Where the person has insight into the changes that are happening to them, especially during the early stages, we need to be alert to signs of depression and seek specialised support early.

13. What is the life expectancy of the person with dementia?

I have not known anyone, who has been correctly diagnosed with dementia and Down syndrome, who has lived longer than five years. Therefore three to four years would appear to be the norm.

14. How is dementia diagnosed?

I particularly like this description on diagnosis of Alzheimer's dementia from Jaber F. Gubrium (gerontologist) and have referred to it many times:

'Diagnostically Alzheimer's is a disease of exclusion. This means when a physician is presented with a possible Alzheimer's patient, he/she engages their investigative work up by ruling out other diseases that may mimic Alzheimer's as a dementia. This basically means looking for other reasons why the person is presenting with dementia-like symptoms. There is a multitude of them. Much of the diagnostic workup then, concerns the use of investigative techniques that will not pinpoint Alzheimer's disease itself but other conditions that may be causing the symptoms of dementia.'

Therefore, there is no single test for most dementias. For many years we thought that tau tangles and beta-amyloid plaques in the brain were an indicator of Alzheimer's. We now know that most individuals with Down syndrome have these tangles from the age of 40 when only about 8% will start showing any signs of dementia.

Other conditions which have similar symptoms to dementia are:

- **Metabolic disorders** such as hypothyroidism and diabetes.
- **Toxicity** can be caused by wrong dosages or mixing drugs incorrectly. For example, people with Down syndrome are particularly susceptible to folic acid abnormalities as a result of taking anti-anticonvulsants.
- **Infections.** The most common are urinary tract and chest infections.
- **Depression.** Many of the symptoms of depression are like those of dementia but are not necessarily considered in people with reduced communication or experiences. See also grief reactions below.
- **Heart Disease,** especially those that cause reduced blood oxygen levels.
- **Poor nutrition** may cause malnutrition and anaemia.
- **Grief reactions.** Bereavement reaction to a significant person or pet dying, changing accommodation recently – this could just be new room in the same house – a key worker, or favoured carer leaving, another resident moving in or leaving, an activity stopping due to a decrease in funding. Remember a grief reaction can be triggered not just by death but also by loss.
- **Environmental changes.** New people in or out, room changes, building changes.
- **Constipation,** which can cause a build-up of toxins within the body resulting in confusion and disorientation.
- **Bone fractures.** Older people with Down syndrome are more susceptible to osteoporosis. The most common problem noted are hip fractures. If an individual is not mobile and has no recognisable way of describing pain, a fracture may go unnoticed and the person's reaction to pain may be mistaken for dementia.
- **Excess alcohol.** Now that many people with learning difficulties are living in less supported and restrictive environments, they, like most people, can make unhealthy choices

that they would have, historically, been denied. Therefore, alcohol consumption should be considered as a possible cause of symptoms.

- **Sensory impairment.** Poor eyesight and hearing loss can lead to social isolation. As discussed earlier, characteristics of Down syndrome include visual and hearing impairments from birth and the ageing process can exacerbate these.

Therefore, for an effective diagnosis to be made an approach involving a multi-disciplinary team, including those the person spends most time with, is essential. The role of relatives and carers are detailed in the answer to the Question 16.

Testing for conditions other than dementia will include a wide variety of background information to be drawn together, e.g. blood tests, brain scans, detailed discussions with those who know the person best, looking for accurate changes to normal behaviour and personality. These tests can take months.

Currently there is a strong argument that for many people with Down syndrome we cannot, with certainty, say they have dementia while they are alive, or afterwards, unless a brain biopsy is performed.

What we can say is that given their symptoms, and ruling out other possible causes, dementia would appear to be present. It is only by brain biopsy after death for most individuals that dementia can be factually confirmed.

15. How does the Mental Capacity Act affect Down syndrome and dementia practice?

This could be a book by itself, but for here I will concentrate on the impact of the five core principles of the Act and comment on a few other areas covered by the Act. For those wanting more technical details after reading this please go to the appendix for relevant website addresses.

For most carers and family members, your practice is already excellent. The 2007 Mental Capacity Act in its five core principles brought together existing good practice and placed them in a legal framework.

Hopefully, for most of the areas I cover here you will be saying, 'But we already do that!' in which case excellent, but I want to make sure you know where your good practice fits into legal requirements.

The five core principles:

1. Assumption of capacity

A person is deemed to have capacity to make a decision unless it is proven otherwise. This means that without a conversation relating to the area where capacity is being assessed you are not assessing capacity.

Let's look at something simple like supporting someone to get up and dressed. A good practice guide for this is to knock on the door and wait, if appropriate, for permission to enter. Enter talking to the person, e.g. 'Good Morning, would you like to get up?' 'Would you like to go to the bathroom?' Ask the person what they would like to wear.

All these types of statements are questions that the answers, whether verbal or non-verbal, will give you an idea what to do next based on the person's wishes, or what their care or support plans say if unable to answer (see point 2). A person is not to be treated as unable to make a decision unless all practicable steps to help them to do so have been taken without success.

2. Every effort should be made to give the person the opportunity to choose

Core principle two is based on choice.

So, in the above option we may *show* the person more than one choice of trousers/skirt and see which one they choose.

Being non-verbal is not an indicator of loss of capacity. Many of you supporting these individuals already know this and have developed good skills in involving them as fully as you can in decision-making.

We legally must use all our knowledge of an individual's communication skills to support them to make their own decisions wherever possible.

3. Able to make unwise decisions

A person is not to be treated as unable to choose just because the choice they make is thought to be unwise.

My personal favourite of the principles: this is the one that allows us to keep our personality and individuality.

Just because we don't agree with a person's decisions, it does not give us the right to automatically overturn it and make them do what we think is the right thing.

If the person can process the information given and understands the consequences of the decision they are making, then their action is with capacity, unless, obviously, it is dangerous to themselves or others. We need to qualify the word dangerous. As a life choice, for instance, an individual may choose to smoke, drink, consume excessive amounts of sugar while having diabetes. These may well be unwise choices, however, if they understand the consequences of those choices and there are no other people put at risk, or conflicting laws, we have no powers to stop them, only a duty to educate and advise.

If, however, the person has an underlying mental health condition and is assessed by a psychiatrist as being psychotic, due to hallucinations or delusions, then the Mental Health Act gives more powers for carers to follow.

4. Best interest

Any act done, or decision made, under the Act for or on behalf of a person who lacks capacity must be done, or made, in their best interests.

Core principal four only comes into play when principles one and two have shown that, at this time, the person is unable to make the decision for themselves.

In this situation, where best interest decisions are being made on the individual's behalf by others, the care/support plans must indicate what carers should do. It should be stressed that, except in emergencies, no best interest decisions should be made by an individual carer. They should be made by a group of people relevant to the decision being made. These decisions require us to consider an individual's previous wishes if they are known.

In order to make a best interest decision it is important to discuss this with the people who 'know them best'. These may include family, other colleagues and relevant members of the multi-disciplinary team.

Please note best interest meetings can be formal and informal.

They range from day-to-day decisions like what to eat, what to wear, when to get up and go to bed and a host of other basic needs, also more complex decisions like medical/surgical needs, where to live and financial decisions.

5. Least restrictive

Before an act is done, or a decision is made, regard must be given as to whether the purpose for which it is needed can be as effectively achieved in a way that is less restrictive of the person's rights and freedom of action.

Every best interest decision should consider the way it is carried out. In planning we must consider the least intrusive option for the person, the one which reduces the impact on the person, such as freedom of movement and individual choice

The above principles often cause confusion when supporting

people who have Down syndrome and dementia, especially as they progress further into their dementia and appear less able to make decisions by themselves.

However, good practice has always indicated we should talk through what we are doing to or for anybody.

In following good practice guidelines, having these conversations and offering choice, we find, especially in the earlier stages of dementia, that people are often able to make more decisions, or parts of decisions, for themselves.

This is good person-centred practice.

A diagnosis of dementia does not, in itself, mean the person lacks capacity.

It does mean that the person will find it increasingly difficult to make decisions, and support to do this will need to be given as the dementia progresses.

Assessing capacity

Probably the most controversial area of the Act within training sessions.

I believe the Act is reasonably clear.

Each decision from the very minor to the major must have a decision-maker who takes responsibility for the decision made.

Guidance states that a decision-maker is the best-placed person and that they must speak to those who know the person best in order to make a safe decision. They must also consider any Advanced Decision (see below) the individual may have made. All those involved are bound by the five core principles.

The decision-maker could be, for example, a family member, support worker, doctor or social worker depending on the decision to be made. You need to be aware of the areas you are responsible for when making decisions.

Advanced decisions

The Mental Capacity Act 2007 put in place legal powers for everyone, with capacity, to have the right to make binding health-care decisions for their future should they lose the ability to make those decisions for themselves at a later date: specifically, end of life decisions such as refusal of resuscitation or medication to preserve life and. Advanced decisions, in almost all situations, are legally binding and should form a large part of any decision made in these areas by the support team and family members.

Lasting Powers of Attorney

The introduction, by the Act, of Lasting Powers of Attorneys, gave everybody with capacity the opportunity to choose who we would like to look after our affairs when we have lost the capacity to do this for ourselves.

The Lasting Power of Attorney for Property and Affairs replaces the old Enduring Power of Attorney and is responsible for financial decisions. The Mental Capacity Act introduced the new Lasting Power of Attorney for Personal Welfare. This person (or people) has the responsibility to make decisions in relation to personal welfare including end of life issues. Both these attorneys can be the same or different people but require separate applications.

Lasting Powers of Attorney are also bound by the five core principles of the Act.

In all areas where disputes cannot be resolved locally, the Court of Protection is the final arbiter of decisions.

For more information on the Mental Capacity Act 2005 please see useful website address in the appendix.

16. How can we help in supplying information that aids diagnosis?

I have heard many critical comments against health care professionals, by carers and family members, at or around the time of diagnosis. Comments like 'They hardly know them', 'They only see them at clinics for a few minutes at a time, how can they make a diagnosis?'

For an accurate diagnosis to be made all those involved with the support and medical care of a person need to communicate effectively with each other. It is the responsibility of each individual and group to help look for and, where appropriate, eliminate other causes of the symptoms.

Whether through lack of confidence or lack of knowledge it would be fair to say that many carers, paid or unpaid, have not always given the professionals, whose responsibility is to diagnose, the information they need to make the best decisions. Therefore, it is not a surprise that, on occasions, diagnosis can be incorrect.

One solution to this problem is ensuring we gather relevant information to inform those involved with the process of diagnosis. For many years I have been suggesting that carers and family members develop the following assessment for everyone with Down syndrome. This assessment should be carried out annually, for anyone over the age of 40, and need be no more than one side of A4 paper.

The assessment is specifically looking at areas where you would be able to see quickly if changes or deterioration occur:

- **Last skill learned** – This could be something as simple as making a cup of tea, making their own bed, road-crossing or tying their own shoelaces, but it needs to be a skill learned and now carried out by the person by themselves. The last skill learned may be one of the first lost during dementia.

- **Idiosyncratic trait** – What makes the person an individual, something they regularly do that is unique to them? For example, a particular, consistent greeting they give to a carer or family member or something that always make them laugh, e.g. at someone else's misfortune, a certain type of sarcasm or requesting something at the same time each day. These differences define individuality.
- **Interest or hobby** – This could be a specific programme on television that is part of their routine, making jigsaws, drawing, writing, even something as simple as copying letters. You are looking at their individual routine and identifying elements they find important to themselves.
- **Fine finger manipulation** – What does the individual do that requires this? For example, tying shoelaces, making a cup of tea/coffee/juice, Makaton, opening a letter, book, buttering toast, riding a bike. This needs to be something the person does by themselves that you would notice them having problems with completing.
- **Memory** – The person goes to the local shop and buys items for themselves, goes to college to attend a course, works part-time in a charity shop, goes to visit a friend or family member by themselves as part of their routine. The important point here is that the activity is carried out with a reasonable level of independence.
- **Non-verbal communication** – Smiling, sighing, waving, being tearful. It doesn't matter what it is, but you can set your clock by it: it always happens in a specific situation.

From the above six areas compile a list of eight to ten points that define the individual, ensuring you, where possible, use all six areas. This is their assessment tool. Review the tool once yearly. Remember to update changes to their routine, e.g. newly learned skill or a new activity that requires memory. If you keep these reviews in chronological order, they will also show the development of the individual. Where more than one area is deteriorating alarm bells should start ringing.

Remember in the first instance your reaction may only need to be contacting opticians, dentists, audiologists or assessing changes in their environment that may be provoking the grief response in the person. However, if the deterioration continues and you need to refer for further assessment just imagine how much more useful professionals may find it if you can provide this assessment and show the areas of change that are present.

At this point it is important to recognise that due to the level of learning disability someone may have, it is not easy, and in some situations almost impossible, to diagnose dementia, especially where the disability is profound and there is no ability to evaluate things such as memory or last skill learned. Remember diagnosis is dependent on change from the norm in a range of areas, so in profound disability, with our current diagnostic tools, for some people a diagnosis of dementia is impossible.

17. How does dementia affect memory?

There are many things that affect our memory, not just dementia. How many of you reading this would agree that your memory is not as good as it used to be? How many of you make lists so that you can remember to complete tasks? How many of you get to the top of the stairs and pause trying to remember what you came up the stairs for? For many of us memory changes are a normal part of ageing but most of us will not develop dementia.

In dementia the changes are more profound, and the deterioration is ongoing.

All memory starts with the five senses, sight, hearing, touch, smell, and taste. Immediate memories are initially stored in our short-term memory and then, in time, are moved to a variety of long-term memory areas within the brain. With the onset of dementia, the first impact is on short-term memories. This is shown when people regularly forget to take medication, an appointment, a name, what day it is, and are more likely to get lost by not recognising local landmarks.

As the dementia progresses, individuals have less access to what is happening now and more to what has happened historically. This 'regression' is because older memories have moved to the foreground in place of more current memories that they cannot retrieve. Therefore, individuals may be communicating about something that they believe to be current while you know the event happened some years ago.

In functional areas, for example urinary continence, we see a change over a period of time. The person does not move overnight from continent to incontinent. It may start with the occasional 'accident' and progress in time to full incontinence. The same is true with mobility.

It is important to note that road safety skills are lost earlier in people with Down syndrome and dementia, than those in the general population who have dementia. The reason for this is not understood. Therefore, risk assessments in this area should be completed at the earliest possible stage and updated regularly.

Despite what many of us think, the fact is that under normal circumstances memories are rarely lost; it is the retrieval systems for these memories that are the problem. This can cause us confusion as some 'retrieval' systems remain intact while others are impaired. For example, it is not uncommon for a person who has dementia, who appears to have forgotten how to speak and communicate effectively, suddenly to be able remember all the words of a song.

18. Do people with Down syndrome age more quickly?

Research continues in this area and we are interested to know the eventual findings. However, the current evidence appears to suggest that, in some areas, people with Down syndrome age faster than the general population.

One area which appears to age more quickly is the brain, presumably because of the extra chromosome 21 present in Down syndrome.

The research has shown that the formation of Alzheimer-like beta-amyloid plaques and tau tangles are found in most people with Down syndrome by the time they reach 40.

It must be emphasised that over 25% of these individuals do not go on to develop Alzheimer's, therefore it is not a diagnostic tool in its own right. (See answer to Question 14.)

Other areas where medical problems occur earlier in people with Down syndrome than the general population include eyes, ears, osteoporosis, menopause and gum disease.

From my own observations of health changes, based on the many people with Down syndrome I have met and discussions with those who support them, in a wide variety of disciplines, there would appear to be premature ageing in areas including hearing, vision and mobility.

In most cases these changes happen around the time that the skin starts to sag. I frequently hear times that the person 'used to have a youthful appearance with tight facial skin' but now they have a very wrinkled appearance and look much older. This normally occurs between 50–60 years old.

Therefore, I recommend that when skin changes become obvious vision and hearing should be assessed even if there are no obvious signs of deterioration.

19. Are some colours an issue for some individuals with dementia?

There is very little research to be found in this area specifically for people with Down syndrome and dementia, so I will draw on examples of stories I have been told or examples I have been involved with. Before you read any further please do not take colour out of anyone's life unless there is a problem you need to react to. The stories below are not the norm but very real to the people involved.

About five years ago I trained a staff team who were supporting a lady with Down syndrome. They suspected her to be developing dementia. The training went well and based on the descriptions given by carers I agreed that dementia was likely to be diagnosed.

About three weeks later I received a distressed call from the manager of the home involved saying that the lady we had discussed had not slept in her room for two nights and was refusing to go into her bedroom.

I agreed to call in the next day. On checking the bedroom, the only eye-catching thing was a beautiful handmade black and white patchwork bed cover, made be a family member. It was striking with very sharp lines which gave it a three-dimensional appearance. We took this cover off and the lady, on being reintroduced into her bedroom, immediately lay down on her bed and there were no further problems in this area.

About seven years ago, while training the team of a residential home, a problem was raised concerning a support worker in the team who was being regularly assaulted by a lady with Down syndrome who had dementia. We discussed this issue and a characteristic of one of the carers emerged: the carer regularly wore an orange mohair cardigan while at work.

I went to visit this home and sat beside the lady concerned. She quickly fell asleep, which did nothing for my ego. The carer, concerned, entered the room wearing her cardigan and within less than a second the resident was awake and obviously agitated, rising from her chair and threatening the carer. We suggested removing the cardigan and the problem disappeared at once.

It was clearly not a problem with the carer but with the interpretation of what she was wearing. I called the manager a few weeks later to be told the problem had not recurred.

I have heard many stories over the years about abnormal reactions to colours. Commonly these include reflective stripes on tracksuit bottoms, coloured plates that some people refuse to eat from and bedroom decorations. However, it must be added that in the majority there are no issues with primary colours and therefore no changes should be made unless problems occur.

20. Is lighting an issue for some individuals with dementia?

Part of the problem here comes from the issues raised in Question 5, specifically eye problems. The Down Syndrome Association have some excellent information on eye problems in adults with Down syndrome. Please see the appendix for Down syndrome website details for those who want more information.

I would rather look at the impact of these problems for the individual and how lighting may play a part in reducing this impact.

During my training and consultancy one of the main symptoms that has been described is that the individual has problems interpreting shadows and lines in carpets or changes of colour on the floor.

This often results in the individual shuffling and stepping over the line or colour in an exaggerated fashion, clearly mis-interpreting the visual image of what is actually there.

This in turn can cause loss of confidence as their environment appears more hazardous than it really is.

Glare is another issue. Stepping into an area where the light is much brighter, for instance into sunshine or from a poorly lit area into a well-lit area.

Neon lights are also often identified as creating difficulties with problems ranging from a potential cause of increase in epileptic activity to increased behavioural problems.

Tips to manage lighting issues

- **Referral to ophthalmic specialists,** to identify and, where possible, use aids to correct or improve the situation.
- **The use of up lighting,** to reduce the number of shadows and glare. This should start in the bedroom, then the areas where the person spends most time.
- **Practical aids,** for example, a wide brimmed hat when moving into sunlight reduces the glare effect, or react-to-light glasses.
- **Talking** a person through a situation where they are showing distress based on how they are visually interpreting their situation.
- **Becoming their eyes** and finding carpet runners, changes in colours before they walk over them.
- **Being aware** that they may not be interpreting the same visual clues as you are, because of actual eye problems, gives you the opportunity to better understand why they may be behaving as they are and to plan how to support more effectively.

21. Are there any communication tips during the early stage of dementia?

In the early stages of dementia, it is so important to involve the person in the changes that are happening to them. This is obviously dependent, to a certain extent, on their ability and activity levels prior to diagnosis.

For many relatives and carers, the main problem is their own denial, a constant wish for the person to get better and return to 'normal'. This too often leads to pushing them to who they were and not accepting where they are going.

Once a diagnosis of dementia is received it is important to ensure we are better informed about the process and how we can best support the individual to maximise their life experiences in a deteriorating situation. There is a lot of living and life to still be enjoyed with a diagnosis of dementia once we better understand and come to terms with reality.

In addition to reading this, please visit the websites identified in the appendix to keep up to date with any advances and advice.

Loss of spontaneous communication

This usually occurs earlier in people with Down syndrome and dementia. This is the normal communication they have with you started by themselves.

For instance, when you arrive at work the individual may have a usual greeting, such as 'How are your family?' or 'What did you do yesterday?'

You know the people you support; you know their communication with you both verbal and non-verbal. Remember this communication is individual and vitally important both to the person and to you. It helps define the individuality of the person.

When the person loses spontaneous communication these conversations and non-verbal communications may just stop. It is important that you continue the conversation as if they had started it; you will often find that they will become involved in the conversation as if they had started it.

For example, if someone asks you how your family are as a normal interaction when you arrive at work, and has stopped asking you, you should start the conversation the way you would if they had asked you how your family were.

If the person is non-verbal but always smiled at you when you came into their space, you should smile back as if they had smiled first.

Sadly, too often what happens is that as the person stops communicating with us we fail to communicate with them, leaving the person isolated and unable to 'step into' a conversation.

Communicating choices

As a result of the changes in short-term memory, offering choices for people with dementia can confuse and cause distress.

An effect of dementia is that with the failure of memory, the person is unable to hold new information and therefore may not be able to process the information that would enable them to make a choice.

I am not suggesting you stop offering choice, but if the individual is becoming more agitated about making choices you need to discuss this and work out how to achieve an outcome that causes the person to become less agitated.

Family and carers will need to rethink their ways of communicating. When previously easy communication is met with confusion, instead of saying 'What would you like to drink?' it is better to say, 'Here is your tea', as you know that this would have been their preferred choice.

If you need to make changes to choice, because the person is finding it difficult, amend the care/support plan accordingly, explaining the areas where and why choice will be reduced and how family members and carers should communicate with the person concerned.

Services that are registered and inspected may be worried that not offering the same level of choice to all the service users could cause concern to monitoring authorities. Therefore, it is important to record carefully why you are working in this way. You may also want to copy this page or print information on the subject from one of the websites listed later, and include it as part of the individual's care/support plan.

The following are other communication tips to consider, which may be relevant to the person you support but remember you need to personalise these to the individual and their needs.

Reorienting

You may on occasion need to reintroduce yourself to the person if they can't remember who you are, especially if you haven't known them for long, or haven't seen them for some time or on a regular basis. This may be especially relevant for domiciliary care workers.

All tasks such as meals, dressing, bathing, toilet needs, going to bed or going out are likely to take more time to explain. You may need to describe what you are going to do, giving verbal and/or visual clues as necessary, while recognising that time-orientating the person is also important, e.g. 'Oh, it's 12.30 pm, do you smell that lovely smell? It's lunchtime,' is much better than calling into a room, 'Lunchtime, come on.'

Using non-verbal communication

As dementia progresses, people begin to lose their ability to verbally communicate and their ability to understand spoken communication diminishes.

However, the ability to understand non-verbal communication remains long after verbal skills are lost. It is therefore vitally important to be even more aware of your own body language. Being friendly, smiling, and having a calm and positive attitude can work wonders when words are not working.

Truth, lie or collusion

See the answer to Question 34.

22. Are there any communication tips as the dementia advances?

When the person moves to the stage of receptive and expressive dysphasia, where they appear to have stopped understanding normal communication, they stop being able to interact verbally, even to well-known and previously well-liked individuals.

It is then that we must move to a sensory level of communication.

Why would you ask someone a complex question when they are unable to carry out even basic tasks? For example, saying, 'What's wrong?' or 'What would you like to do today?'

I am not suggesting we should never say these things; they are after all facets of good practice and normal communication; it is still important to talk our way through our interactions and involve the individual as much as possible.

However, we should be prepared for the person not to answer in any meaningful form. They are not being awkward or cantankerous; they are unable to process information received and deal with it in a normal fashion.

We need to become more detective-like in our approach, looking for non-verbal clues which might give us more information. You are already aware that the vast percentage of normal communication is non-verbal. As the person you support loses the ability to verbally inform us of their needs, we need to fine tune our reading of this non-verbal communication.

'Would you like to go for a walk in the garden?' may be met with total silence. However, saying brightly, 'Let's go for a walk in the garden', supporting them to get up and walking to the garden may result in the person smiling when they get there.

Our mood, our attitude and how we go about our job is vitally important for good communication in dementia care.

Showing frustration, being under the weather, trying to rush the person through a task and giving confusing messages are all picked up by the person with dementia and will add to their level of stress and anxiety.

We need to become aware of our own non-verbal communication when working with the individual as their dementia is advancing, and always support the person with dignity and respect.

Smiling should never be underestimated – it alone is often reassuring. I remember when my mother-in-law's dementia was advanced, and she had stopped communicating with us as relatives. Many times when I visited her in the nursing home and she was clearly agitated I didn't ask her 'What's wrong?' I merely said don't worry about that, your daughter is sorting that out. The number of times she sighed and calmed down was amazing. I have no reason to believe she understood the words I was saying but do believe she was feeding off my non-verbal com-munication, which included smiling and calm reassurance.

23. What are the signs of dementia as it progresses?

Question 12 covered the early warning signs, now let's look at the signs in the mid and later stages of dementia for the person with Down syndrome.

During the mid-stage

Increased loss of mobility. Moving towards immobility, shuffling gate, being less keen to walk in shaded and bright areas, requiring increased support in all mobility areas.

Depression. As dementia advances, particularly in those individuals with awareness of their deterioration, be aware of rapid flattening of mood, tearfulness, increased confusion and upset about what they can no longer do. Where these symptoms are present refer for psychiatric assessment. Depression is treatable.

Hallucinations. These can affect any of the five senses but the most common are auditory (hearing voices) and visual (seeing things we cannot). Again, knowledge of the individual is important here. Did they always have imaginary friends or foes they communicated with? Could it be agnosia? Agnosia is the loss of ability to accurately recognise objects, faces, voices or places; it can affect all five senses. This is most common in vascular dementia but can be present in other dementias.

Swearing. Especially where the individual would appear to have never sworn and then starts to, this can be alarming to family and carers.

Remember in dementia inhibitions are lowered. Swearing is on TV, radio, in films and heard by most people in society. Hit your thumb with a hammer (accidentality), stub your toe painfully and see how close to swearing most non-swearers come. Swearing is a common reaction to pain and fear.

Irrational fears. The most common ones I have seen and heard about are fear of hair-washing, almost agoraphobic reactions to going outside and problems with colours and lighting (see Questions 19 and 20).

These are not common. I remember one individual who was refusing to go to the bathroom for bathing and hair-washing. Carers described her reaction to these procedures, especially hair-washing, as alarming where she appeared to be terrified.

We discussed separating out these activities as she had previously loved her bath. This worked and she went back to loving her bath-time.

Her hair needs were catered for in a different area from the bathroom, using a mixture of dry shampoos, sponge dampening and reducing the number of times her hair needed to be washed.

We can become obsessive about routines like this, which is unhelpful in good person-centred care.

Always ask yourselves, particularly when a person becomes agitated or resistant:

Why does the task need to be done? How can we do it humanely?

Just because it's Tuesday and that's bath night is not a good enough reason. So be creative in your approach.

Verbal and physical aggression. See answer to Question 26.

Increasing incontinence. Both urinary and faecal. Moving towards accidents becoming the new norm.

Swallowing difficulties. Some of the characteristics of Down syndrome are the tongue being disproportionally large for a small mouth. As dementia progresses the changes that are taking place in the brain can result in the person forgetting how to chew and eat properly. This leads to increased risk of swallowing difficulties and choking.

The experts in this field are speech and language therapists and should be involved as problems are identified.

Increased levels of self-neglect. As the person loses their ability to care for themselves, we see a reduction in the person's hygiene and self-care. This is especially difficult to see when the person was always smart and tidy. We need to take responsibility for supporting and helping people in some of these areas depending on the individual needs of the person.

For example, someone who enjoys makeup may have lost the skills to do this for themselves. This does not necessarily mean they no longer like makeup but need more help than they did before.

During the later stage

Weight Loss. Problems with the digestive system absorbing the nutrition from their diet, problems with the reducing appetite of the individual with dementia, problems with how the food is presented, e.g. a soft/liquidised diet, can all combine to encourage weight loss. (See Question 24.)

Self-neglect. Now fully dependant on family and carers carrying out all personal care for the individual.

Malnutrition. See weight loss above and Question 24.

Double incontinence. Total urinary and faecal incontinence.

Receptive and expressive dysphasia. The individual not appearing to be involved in receiving or giving any communication relevant to their current situation.

General slowing down towards the end of life. Most of the time the person is now appearing unresponsive, with increasing respiratory and circulation problems. Family and carers following an end of life plan for the individual.

Tremor. Shaking in the hands, sometimes more general body shakes.

Epileptic seizures. A small group of people develop epileptic activity towards the end of their life.

Immobility This is now total, with mobility skills lost. For many this happens in the mid-stages, but is the new normal in the end stage.

24. How important is a good diet for the individual with dementia?

The most important and underheard statement is 'We are what we eat and drink'. A balanced diet. What is it? What does it look like?

If we are truly into person-centred care, then this surely means the diet that is the most suitable and needed by the individual.

I have trained and worked with nutritionists and dieticians over the years and learned from them that there is no set foods or menus for the person with dementia. Rather there is personal taste and what a person will tolerate.

Let's look at one common complaint that has been raised by almost every group during training: 'We offer drinks on a regular basis, but the person won't drink enough.' We must, therefore, think outside the box; that is what person-centred requires.

Try food with lots of fluid in them. It is hard to refuse a wet slice of cantaloupe melon for most people. Or what about a milkshake, jellies or a spoonful of fresh fruit salad?

Both in dementia and ageing we see a reduction of taste buds and therefore need to compensate with increasing flavour. Using seasoning like all spice can lift flavour and make food more enjoyable. Garlic, ginger, chilli and turmeric can not only lift flavour and appearance but also have additional health benefits.

Please taste, seeking appropriate permissions first, what you are giving to see if you would want to eat it. For example, have you ever tasted drinks or other food substitutes where the person requires soft food due to swallowing problems? Can you add some fresh fruit juice?

There is evidence in dementia of not only reduced taste buds but of reduced appetite when mobility problems increase and activity decreases; therefore, big meals may not be wanted. A general principle is to offer 'little and often'. Many times people will prefer to graze throughout the day.

As co-ordination is deteriorating, does the individual need to use a knife and fork when these are proving difficult for them? Do we take over and feed the person or would it be better to offer finger foods that the person can manage themselves, and thereby maintain their independence for as long as possible?

Sitting with someone and encouraging them by repeatedly reminding them to 'pick up and eat' another piece of food may take a long time but helping to maintain dignity and independence is far more important and rewarding than rushing on to the next task.

Has your service access to a dietician who can assist/advise in the planning of a person-centred diet to help meet the individual's needs? They are the specialists in this area and worth their weight in gold if used properly.

Also consider how we can approach other health issues using food, one example being when systems slow down as a result of age and immobility. Do people require laxatives to help them, or would it be possible to increase the amount of roughage in their diet?

If sleeping is becoming a problem, are we still supporting someone to have a caffeine drink before they go to bed or should we be encouraging caffeine-free alternatives?

Do not forget some of the old wives' tales work for some people. Many people still use a small glass of sherry before a meal to help prepare the digestive system for food.

25. Is there any medication for dementia?

Although there is no cure for Alzheimer's disease there are medications used to delay the symptoms and slow the progression of the dementia.

Medication such as donepezil have been shown to be effective in people with Down syndrome and dementia. (Professor Andre Strydom of Kings College London. Published in the British Journal of Psychiatry 2017.)

Early diagnosis becomes even more important if medication is to be considered. Medication should be given at a time where it helps the person to maintain skills and decision-making.

People with Down syndrome and dementia may also suffer from other medical and mental health conditions.

These may include conditions such as epilepsy, hypo-thyroidism, chest and other types of infections, heart conditions, bowel problems and then more generally other conditions present in the wider community.

It is therefore not uncommon for an individual to be taking multiple medications.

Do you know the side effects of each individual medication and how these interact with other medications the person may be taking? You should always get a patient information leaflet with all medications, containing information about the medication along with any side effects the person may experience. Please ask the pharmacist if there are any other side effects as a result of the combination of medications being taken. Is there a regular medication review in place? If not, book one in.

Some behaviours are caused by the medication individuals are taking. For example, medication used for constipation often cause stomach pains/cramps. If you have dementia and are already confused and disorientated, how might you react to the pains? (See Question 24 on nutrition.) Many medications used to control behaviour cause restlessness and agitation.

Question 27 looks at medication used for controlling aggression.

Questions 26-32 deal with behaviours that are sometimes seen in dementia and Down syndrome.

You may be familiar with the term 'Challenging Behaviour'. Please never use this term again. Today many people are defined by this term and not enough time is spent recognising that what is happening is a form of communication with us, which we are not understanding.

This does not usually need a specialist team. It can normally be done by families and carers spending time to look beyond the behaviour to the emotion that may be causing it.

Using the term 'behaviour that challenges us to understand' is an excellent way of seeing things differently. Using this description puts the responsibility back on us to find out why the behaviour is happening.

We recognise that all behaviour is a form of communication. When someone smiles or laughs, we know they are communicating joy; when they cry, we know they are unhappy.

If we take this knowledge into examining negative behaviours, we will better understand its reasons and in some cases resolve it or, if needed, involve specialist teams earlier.

The 2014 Care Act set out the reporting procedures for us all to follow if we suspect abuse of a person at risk. Many referrals are made each year in this area either because of the way carers or families are working with individuals or because of the impact of behaviour on other service users. It is a legal responsibility to report any suspected abuse you may witness to the local authority safeguarding teams via your procedures.

For staff working in services regulated by the Care Quality Commission please read further information on positive behaviour support available on their website. Also remember your requirements as set out in Regulations 9, 12, 13,17 and 18. In addition, the requirements of the Mental Health Act code of practice, 2005 Mental Capacity Act and NICE guideline 10.

26. Why do some individuals with dementia become aggressive?

Please find listed below a variety of reasons why some people may become aggressive and apply this list to each incident as a means of finding out why this behaviour may be occurring.

A person's usual way of coping with stress

This is now emphasised and regarded as a problem.

Before dementia, was the person someone who reacted aggressively to situations? Did they stamp their feet when upset? Were they naturally impatient? How did they cope when frustrated?

The effect of dementia usually reduces normal inhibitions. Control mechanisms can be lowered so the person expresses themselves in a cruder way.

Ensure you are taking the person's historical personality traits into account when investigating behaviours

Assertion of will or attempt to sustain dignity

I want to paint you a picture and see how you may react.

You are a proud, dignified person. You look after all your own personal needs including your toilet needs well.

You have now developed dementia and are losing control of your bladder.

You are sitting in your chair and your bladder has just emptied. A stranger comes and supports you to the toilet, they talk to you and explain what they are doing but you don't really understand what they are saying. Your clothes are removed. This stranger now starts to wash and clean you between your legs.

How might you be feeling at this moment? How might you react?

The above example covers issues such as coping with embarrassment, not interpreting normal communication well, people wanting you to do things when you are already busy doing something else, carers being task-orientated and rushing you when you don't really understand what is happening, carers talking to each other and ignoring you while they violate your privacy.

Response to unmet need

When memory is failing, and a person has forgotten how to communicate effectively, people may act in inappropriate ways to get their needs met. Some of the needs that often cause a negative reaction are:

Pain (toothache, stomach cramps, headache are some examples), hunger, thirst, toilet needs, boredom, wanting to be somewhere else because you don't know where you are, wanting to be with a family member or carer who you have forgotten is no longer around, believing you should be somewhere else because your current memories do not match where you are now.

Response to the environment

What is happening in the environment? Noise, smells, other people, what are they doing? Are there issues with lighting or colours? Is the current environment unfamiliar?

I remember supporting John, who had Down syndrome and dementia.

He lived in a home for people with learning difficulties in Leicester. Before developing dementia, his parents visited regularly to take him home every weekend, a 120-mile round trip for them.

John's dad sadly died, and his mum moved closer to John's location. He still went home every weekend to Mum's new house.

John then developed dementia and after a short period of time started having problems when Mum took him home.

It became clear that John's regression within his dementia no longer allowed him to recognise Mum's new home: he was looking for the environment he was used to in the family home 60 miles away. After a short period of time Mum only visited John in his home and stopped taking him to an environment that caused him confusion and made him feel anxious and uncomfortable.

Reaction to failure

This can happen especially in the early stages where the person is more aware of their recent past and therefore may be more aware of the changes that are happening to them. Remember a normal mental health mechanism in this situation is denial; we must learn to deal with this denial sympathetically and not just challenge it.

For example, when some people start to become incontinent of urine, they may blame someone else rather than accept it was them. This denial is often due in part to frustration and embarrassment that they wet themselves. A common reaction by family members and carers is to say, 'Why didn't you tell me that you needed the toilet?' A better response may be to say, 'Come on and we will sort that out.' The second response casts no blame on the individual.

A real frustration for carers is that the person may meet their own toilet needs sometimes and at other times be incontinent. There is often a belief that this may be manipulative, attention-seeking behaviour and therefore challenge the person.

In dementia, where a person has had no earlier issues in this area, these, at first occasional, accidents are part of the normal deterioration and holding the person to account is cruel and more likely to lead to inappropriate behaviours.

Response to unresolved emotional trauma

Do we know the histories of the people we support? Were they at any point in their lives left bereaved, moved into the care of others, bullied, abused or unhappy?

What if the person regresses to a period of their life where this was happening? How might they be feeling?

How might they react differently to, say, intimate care?

It would be useful if each person, before they develop other conditions, had a single sheet of significant dates throughout their lives. This should include significant traumatic events in their lives in chronological order.

Frustration

This is caused by a realisation of a growing disability or loss. Remember depression is a normal reaction to growing disability and loss. We are always affected when we are working with/ supporting someone with dementia, especially when we knew them before they developed this condition. We talk about the personality being stripped away in front of our eyes. How much worse is this for the person, especially if they are retaining some insight into their deterioration? Depression should have already been checked for before it is agreed that dementia is present (see Question 14). Once dementia has been diagnosed, we need to be alert for the symptoms of depression as deterioration continues. Depression can and should be treated if present.

27. Does medication used to control aggression work?

A Department of Health paper entitled 'Quality outcomes for people with dementia: building on the work of the National Dementia Strategy', published 8 September 2010 (see Appendix), states on page 10:

'**Reduced use of antipsychotic medication** – There are an estimated 180,000 people with dementia on antipsychotic drugs. In only about one third of these cases are the drugs having a beneficial effect and there are 1,800 excess deaths per year as a result of their prescription.' This paper also recommended a reduction of two thirds in the use of antipsychotic medication over a period of two years.

Clearly, dementia is a psychosis. A psychosis is a major mental disorder where people lose some contact with reality. This might involve seeing or hearing things that other people cannot see or hear (hallucinations) and believing things that are not actually true (delusions). In some cases, medication is appropriate and necessary, e.g. controlling hallucinations, extreme aggression, inappropriate behaviours.

It is important to remember that for a person with dementia, not being in the 'here and now' is rarely a psychotic reaction.

Most of the people I have supported who have lost contact with reality have regressed and their orientation to time and place is the issue, not a psychosis.

Another name for antipsychotic drugs is major tranquilisers. They aim to eliminate or reduce the intensity of certain symptoms, e.g. aggression. When you see the list of possible side effects of antipsychotic drugs listed below you will understand why they should only be used as a last resort, after other non-drug approaches have failed, and should be regularly reviewed every 6–12 weeks.

Possible side effects of antipsychotics include:

- Sedation (drowsiness)
- Parkinsonism (shaking and unsteadiness)
- Increased risk of infections
- Increased risk of falls
- Increased risk of blood clots
- Increased risk of ankle swelling
- Increased risk of stroke
- Worsening of other symptoms of dementia
- Increased risk of death

(Side effects taken from the Alzheimer's Society website: Anti-psychotic Drugs.)

28. Are there other ways to control aggression other than medication?

All forms of aggression are unacceptable, and we must have a zero tolerance towards them. I have never seen a job description that says being assaulted, spat at or being sworn at is part of the job.

However, I have met many carers who seem to accept such behaviour as the norm within their workplace. When I ask why the behaviour is occurring, I often receive answers like, 'They have always been like that', 'They have got challenging behaviour', or 'They have dementia.'

Never stop asking: 'why?' There is always a reason, even if finding it may seem impossible. It is your job to never give up trying to find out reasons or trying to find solutions that change the severity of the issue.

Risk assessments are crucial to developing good practice. Ask yourselves, what have we learned from each incident? What can we change?

What you need to ask yourselves is why are we referring individuals to their doctor where aggression is the main presenting factor? Have we looked thoroughly into why the person is behaving in this way? Are there any triggers that we can prevent from happening again? Are we seeing the behaviour as a means of communication and spending time to work out what the person is trying to communicate, e.g. pain, dignity, frustration? Use a positive behaviour support approach.

Have you been completing ABC charts to try to understand the behaviour?

Although there are pre-printed ABC charts available you can easily make your own. On a blank sheet of paper draw three columns.

Write the words Antecedence, Behaviour and Consequences, or Before, During, After, as headings in each column. Note, if this is being done in a workplace, also make sure you have left a space for date and name of person completing the form.

Each time the behaviour you are wishing to find causes for occurs, everybody present at the time should individually complete an ABC. Please do not collude or complete as a group as everybody observes things their own way and a vital piece of the 'jigsaw' may be missed, as in a group teams are prone to look for consensus not individuality.

The information you should be recording is:

Antecedence
What happened before the behaviour? Time, place, who else was there, what was happening in the environment, smells, sound, heat, sunlight – anything you think was relevant. What was the person or anyone else saying or doing?

Behaviour
What happened? Describe the incident exactly as it happened.

What words and non-verbal communication occurred? How was the behaviour managed, both by those present and the person themselves?

If anybody was hurt, were they targeted or was it an accident, e.g. was someone in their way as they tried to get out of the room?

How and, if possible, why did the behaviour stop?

It is vitally important to be honest and factual about the incident, and not get caught up in blame or excuses. This can be very difficult if you were involved in the incident

Consequence
How and, if possible, why did the behaviour stop? Was anyone hurt? Did that person or anyone else say or do anything?

Most importantly, was there anything learned from the antecedence or the behaviour that you can address to make the behaviour less likely to happen again? What do you need to do differently?

The ABC system should also be seen as one form of debriefing and done as soon after the incident as possible. You may need to do this on several occasions to see a pattern occurring, like mealtimes, a specific person being assaulted, it always happening before going to bed, etc.

As family members and carers, we must prepare information for clinical staff in a professional manner and constantly look for reasons for such behaviour. The use of ABC charts helps this process.

I believe strongly that many individuals who are assaulted by someone with dementia, physically or verbally, have in some way, albeit accidentally, contributed to the assault themselves by the way they interacted with the person.

This could be anything from attitude, speed of interaction, failure to properly involve the person or offering too many choices, to seeing the task as more important than the person and not respecting the dignity of the person.

The best way to deflect inappropriate behaviour is to spot the early warning signs and then use distraction and diffusion techniques to move the person beyond the behaviour before it becomes a problem.

Here are four short case studies to illustrate this.

- On a Tuesday and Wednesday morning Bill tries to leave the house. When carers intervene, trying to persuade him to stay in, he becomes agitated and distressed.

   You know that in the past these were the two days he used to work at the local garden centre.

   To try and prevent him from becoming agitated his carers, on wakening Bill on Tuesday and Wednesday mornings, talk to him about his job. Does he miss going there? What did he used to do there? Is there anyone he misses? At breakfast they talk to Bill about an activity they know he likes and arrange to do it that morning.
- Jean becomes upset and agitated when the noise level is high. Two other residents in her home are having an argument, nothing serious, but you notice Jean is reacting to the noise. The care plan describes how at these times the

carers should ask Jean if she would like a coffee and encourage her to support them to make it, taking her away from the noise. This frequently works and Jean returns to her usual placid self quickly.

- Ahmed is often agitated during mealtimes, often failing to finish his meal; his carers think it is the hustle and bustle he is reacting to. As the philosophy in the home where he lives is person-centred good dementia care, everybody is supported to eat and drink when and where they want. They often graze little and often and enjoy fewer formal mealtimes, large helpings with groups of others.

- As a result of this Ahmed is eating and drinking when he wants to and not necessarily to our timetable.

In person-centred practice the individual dictates what they want: when, where and with whom. We often fail people when we try to make them follow our routines and rituals. How many of us today sit at a dining table at set times for all our meals? Not many.

For Ahmed, adapting the routine to meet his needs makes eating a more pleasurable, and therefore a more beneficial, experience.

- Rebecca has a habit of pulling the carer's hair when they are working closely with her.

This is especially a problem when they are supporting her to get dressed. They have used ABC charts to try and establish reasons for this behaviour, but can find no explanation for it. It has therefore been agreed that by occupying her hands during this time, e.g. giving her a tennis ball or a ball of wool to hold, she is distracted and less likely to pull hair. In addition, they have risk assessed this situation and agreed that there should be two carers involved: one who distracts Rebecca while the other supports her to dress.

As was the case for Rebecca, in many situations the reason for the behaviour is not obvious or has not yet been found. It is therefore often down to our innovation to devise ways to minimise the behaviour both in frequency and severity.

At all times when we devise strategies to eliminate or reduce behaviours, we must do this in accordance with the requirements of the Mental Capacity Act. The strategies should be recorded as good practice for that individual in that situation. They must never be unilateral acts but agreed with the whole team, and where necessary involve external bodies, for example the local community learning disability team (CLDT).

29. Why do some people with dementia walk purposefully?

There are a variety of logical and explainable reasons purposeful walking occurs. These include:

The person's usual way of coping with stress in the past

How many of us just enjoy going for a walk? If under stress how many of us find a walk reduces our stress? If we recognise that stress is one of the reasons for purposeful walking, then what is causing the stress?

Could stress be caused by hunger, thirst, pain, toilet needs, confusion as to where they are or not recognising others around them?

Searching for security

This can occur when a person is unsure where they are, trying to find something or someone familiar.

Has the person regressed to a point where an event should be happening at that time, for example going to work, a club, a college course?

Response to boredom and low stimulation

Dementia does not mean life stops, rather it continues at a slower pace and should now be geared to maximising quality of life.

Targeting activities that are within the individual's known skill set, at a level where involvement of the individual is encouraged.

Also remember the importance of fixed activities that are essential to normal living. These include, for example, mealtimes, toilet and bathing needs, hair and makeup needs, dressing and undressing, drinks and chatting.

Response to over stimulation

While boredom can lead to one set of problems, doing too much can cause another. This is where true person-centred care and support comes in.

What is the right level of activity for the individual today?

How they are will often be the clue to over or under-stimulation. Read their verbal and non-verbal clues.

I remember the story of a woman from Bristol, who I'll call Gina. Gina had Down syndrome and dementia. Throughout Gina's life one of the most important activities for her was going to the Hippodrome Theatre to watch plays and shows.

Gina's carers supported her in this for many years, helping her to buy tickets and going with her to the theatre.

However, after Gina developed dementia, this became problematic. Although still enjoying going to the theatre she often, after the interval, became tired and agitated, shouting that she wanted to go home. Obviously in addition to Gina's distress it was also affecting other customers' enjoyment and so, sadly, Gina stopped going.

This was someone who loved the theatre and often talked for

weeks after each performance about what she had seen and would go through the programme with carers on many occasions, until the next show.

I was involved in a training session with the carers when they told me this story.

I suggested they contact the theatre about a special ticket for Gina whereby she could go for the first half of the show one night/matinee and then go later to see the second half on another night/matinee.

The theatre bent over backwards to help, offering not only a special ticket price but also sending out the programme to Gina as soon as it was available to them. For the next eight months Gina was able to attend and enjoy the theatre thanks to the carers', and theatre's, innovative approach.

Concentration does not stop when an individual develops dementia, but it will probably be lower.

Eventually Gina stopped going to the theatre on her terms as her visual and hearing problems increased and she no longer enjoyed the experience.

Reaction to prolonged use of some medications

For example, many different medications, including those given to control inappropriate behaviour, have side effects including restlessness and agitation.

30. How do we support someone who walks purposefully?

When is it happening? Does it coincide with anything else that is happening to the individual or the environment?

ABC recording may be useful in identifying patterns to help understand better what may be happening for the individual.

Who is being affected by the behaviour?

Is the person becoming exhausted or losing too much weight?

Is where they are trying to go causing a problem?

We need to assess if the walking is causing a problem. If it is not then why are we concerned? Clearly if it is causing a problem for the person or others we need to be creative as to how we support the situation.

Case study: John

John always becomes restless around 9.30 am, walking to the door and trying to go out. He becomes agitated with his carers, who constantly try to support him back to his seat. On a couple of occasions, he has tried to force his way out and the carers have had to use all their powers of distraction to prevent him from leaving.

This does not happen every day. The care team discover that ten years ago John used to work in a charity shop from 10 am to 1 pm, Monday through to Wednesday. When they check the ABC records, they establish that almost all incidents occurred on these days.

Now that they may have explained why John is more restless and is walking purposefully to the door on these mornings, they are much more likely to be more empathetic to John's needs.

They could, if John is able, talk to him about his time working there. It may be possible to arrange a visit from a carer from the team who used to work with him. They could possibly arrange a visit to the shop if this was agreed as being suitable.

In addition, they should, on Monday–Wednesday mornings at 9.30 am develop an activity that John would like to be involved in to distract him from needing to go out.

Case study: Sonia

Sonia becomes agitated every Sunday at around 11 am.

She is purposefully walking for up to four hours at a time and no matter what the care team do she only sits down at about 3 pm.

She will not eat her lunch but eats well after she has become more settled.

Sonia only moved to her current home two years ago and the team can't understand her behaviour.

They contact someone who used to work with Sonia and has known her for fifteen years. After talking to them about the current concerns the team discover that Sonia's mum always visited on a Sunday morning, stayed for lunch and left about 3 pm.

Sadly, Mum died about six years ago and Sonia struggled with this for about eight months until she finally accepted her mum had died.

They now have a greater understanding of why Sonia may be behaving as she is.

What can be done with this information?

Firstly, let the rest of the team know. Then plan for Sunday in a different way. Recognise that Sonia may have regressed to a time where, in her mind, her mum is still alive, and she is waiting for her.

A few things that could be tried are:

On Sunday morning arrange for Sonia to have one-to-one time. This may distract her memory.

When she first starts to become distressed, intervene, try distraction to an activity you know she likes.

If Mum used to sit beside her for lunch, try having a member of the care team sit beside her for lunch.

Put on a film you know Sonia likes before or after lunch.

Keep trying, but only one thing at a time. It is important to try new things one at a time so you can find out what works.

As said earlier, solutions to problems are rarely found in medication, but rather are far more likely, and safely, found in innovation, creative thinking and not giving up.

If we ever stop asking why a behaviour is happening it may be time to consider alternative employment. I always recommend working in a supermarket because tins don't mind, people do!

31. Why do some people with dementia show inappropriate sexual behaviours?

It is important to remember that as with aggression there should be zero tolerance of inappropriate sexual behaviour, ranging from inappropriate touching to inappropriate conversation.

There are a lot of logical and explainable reasons why sexually inappropriate behaviours occur. These include:

Amplification of earlier sexual conversation/behaviour

- What was their behaviour like in this area before they developed dementia?
- Did they recognise and respect personal space?
- Did they ask for a hug on occasions? How was this normally reacted to?
- How did they express their sexuality?
- Were there any recorded problems in this area?

- What was their conversation like? Was it in any way flirtatious? How was this reacted to?
- Have they had or are they currently in a relationship?

Appropriate urges and inappropriate responses

- What was their previous sexually awareness?
- Are they confusing a carer/service user with a previous partner?
- Did they normally masturbate in the privacy of their room but are now doing so in a non-private area?
- Are certain perfumes, items of clothing, for example, reminding them of a previous partner?

Wish/desire/need for close/intimate contact

- Acting on wishes and needs inappropriately, due to agnosia or loss of inhibition.
- Has the person always been a 'touchy feely' individual? Not a respecter of personal space?

Agnosia is common in dementia. It is a problem with recognition affecting any of the five senses. In this situation it is usually visual, where a person sees someone other than the person in front of them, perhaps an ex-partner or someone they shared intimacies with. It could be set off by the smell of a specific perfume, clothing or similar physical appearance.

Previous institutional care

Personal space issues are managed differently today as compared to the norm within institutional care. There, personal space issues were often not a key issue as this was a group that was isolated from society and therefore hugging and poor respecting of personal space was common.

It may be as simple as someone who spent many years in the

institution regressing to that time and doing what was accepted as normal. For example, when I started my career in the learning disability field in the early 1980s it was not uncommon to see an adult, who had Down syndrome, sitting on a member of staff's knee.

Misunderstanding when personal care is being given

As a result of agnosia or because of confusion and disorientation in time and place some people with dementia misunderstand intimate personal care or even friendly approaches inside their personal space to be sexual advances and respond accordingly.

32. How should we support individuals who show inappropriate sexual behaviours?

As with other behaviours, the use of ABC charts often prove useful here in identifying why the behaviour may be happening. The better your knowledge of the person before they developed dementia the greater the accuracy in identifying the problem.

It may be as simple as someone who spent many years in the institution regressing to that time and doing what was accepted as normal.

Where there is a problem causing issues for the person themselves or others there is a need to develop clear management procedures.

I trained as a sexual health enabler back in the early 1990s and have found many occasions where individuals are carrying out natural behaviour that is upsetting the care team only.

For example, masturbation is a natural activity and where it is carried out safely, in privacy, it should not be seen as a problem. Our value base should not determine how individuals should behave.

Unfortunately, many people with a learning difficulty live their lives in a goldfish bowl with all aspects of their behaviour more easily visible. We need to ensure safe spaces are available when someone is behaving inappropriately in more public spaces.

Most carers and family members are not experts in this field and therefore managing inappropriate sexual behaviour should involve referral to psychologists, sexual health therapists or other specifically qualified professionals for advice and guidance.

Care teams should follow policy and guidance on dress code and makeup to ensure they are not increasing the risk for themselves.

Occasionally someone raises the issue of a service user who accuses carers of sexually inappropriate behaviour on a regular basis, which after investigation proves to be false; this is very rare. It is important that the risk assessment should give clear guidance as to how to provide support to the person: for example, should there be more than one carer providing support for the individual, maybe even including things like which gender of staff should offer support.

Obviously the first time these types of allegations are made they should be properly investigated, and if discovered to be unfounded and the allegations continue you should evaluate:

What did we learn from the first time?

How do we change how we are working to ensure both the individual and care team are safe?

In all these types of situations expert support should be gained from safeguarding teams and appropriate sexual health professionals. This should be reflected in the paperwork.

33. How can you support someone who asks cyclical/repetitive questions?

This is one of the more common questions raised.

Care home teams, especially, will ask how to deal with someone who repeatedly asks who is coming on the next shift, 20 to 30 times a shift.

It is important to note that people with dementia who ask repetitive questions do not ask 'repetitive questions'. Every time they ask you the question it is the first time they have asked it, as their loss of short-term memory does not allow them to remember they have already asked it.

Carers need to learn coping strategies, not penalise the person for asking the question for the first time, even if it is the twentieth time it has been answered.

When I faced this issue as a clinical manager, we turned this into a game for the team. We produced ten possible ways of answering the question to give us variety and challenge us as a team to become less frustrated.

Answers could include the following sequence.

Giving the names of carers coming on the next shift. Giving photos of who is coming on next. Asking the person who they think is coming on next. Asking the person to look in their pocket to see the pictures of who is coming on the next shift.

Remember our non-verbal communication of impatience; throwing our eyes up, tone of voice and facial frustration may confuse and agitate the individual.

34. Should you collude/agree with someone with dementia when you know they are wrong?

I approach this question from a humanitarian point of view.

Should we continually bring a person back to reality when the consequence of doing this is to cause them pain?

Let me give you an example of this from the mainstream area, from my own clinical practice, to show you what I mean.

An elderly lady with dementia, living in a nursing home, wakes each morning and says to the carers that she needs to go downstairs, despite living in ground floor accommodation, to make breakfast for her children.

The carers gently remind her each morning that her children died some years ago in a tragic car accident.

This shows her different reality where she believes she is in a different location, in a different time. As a result of the carer's interaction, this lady each morning goes into a grief wheel, becoming very upset and tearful lasting for 20 minutes or more until she appears to forget why she was upset.

As a new manager we discussed this situation. The carers told me they were unhappy about this as well but the previous manager was a reality-orientation purist believing that our job was to bring people back into reality when they 'slipped out'.

We decided that we would reply to her request to go downstairs to make breakfast for her children by saying to her, 'well we will see you downstairs then.' This worked perfectly, as by the time we got to the dining room she had forgotten about them. We never had to wake her painfully again.

However, we have an ethical duty not to lie intentionally. I see most of the good work in this area as being distraction rather than deception and good recording, which allows others to understand our approach in these situations.

35. What activities are useful for people with Down syndrome and dementia?

It is important to first look at the purpose of activity. Words that come to my mind include stimulation, motivation, contact, bonding (however brief), connecting, bringing back memories, usefulness, occupation, purpose and reality. What works best for the individual is something they want to do at that time that is already in their skill set.

This is where previous knowledge of the individual becomes very important. People with dementia have great difficulty when asked to learn new skills.

At all stages of dementia, you are hoping to enhance the individual's quality of life and encourage their involvement, however brief or small that may be.

Activities do not need to be set to specific times of the day or days of the week, instead they should take place when the individual is most receptive to them. Most activities are therefore individual to the person's timetable.

Each person should have a list of activities that they enjoy and find in any way stimulating. This list should be continually updated as the person moves through their dementia.

I have lost count of the times I have heard, from carers, 'We don't have the time for activities. We are too busy.'

I first heard this back in the late 1980s when I was managing a forty-bedded care of the elderly unit for people with learning disabilities in a long-stay institution. I didn't agree with it then and I still don't now.

Look at all the tasks that are necessary for us to be involved in to maintain a good quality of life for those we care for. Supporting dressing, mealtimes, toilet/bathing needs, for example, are all one-to-one time.

How are we using that time? Are we interacting, encouraging participation, comforting, telling stories and encouraging communication?

A task is never just a means to an end; it is also an opportunity for communication and two-way involvement.

It has become more popular in many care homes to employ activity coordinators. Having now met with many of them they, when used appropriately, are a valuable addition to any team.

Many of them agree that set activities on a set timetable rarely work because of the diverse needs of the group and how lucid and 'present' the individuals are at any given time.

Those who are operating a high level of good practice say they give the opportunity for individuals to be involved in an activity they are known to like, and interact with them when they are taking part. So, at any one time one person may be drawing on paper while another is looking at a magazine and yet another is looking through a family photograph album.

Some activities can, if well managed, be communal. Mainly in the areas of music and movement. Many people enjoy singing or listening and moving to music.

However, despite the benefit of having an activity coordinator, it is every carer's responsibility to ensure they are offering activity opportunities to the people they care for, no matter how advanced their dementia is.

An activity is anything that stimulates and involves a person for any length time, however long or brief, from peeling potatoes to knitting, from helping get dressed to helping washing their hands, from planting flowers to buttering their own bread, from enjoying having their makeup put on to enjoying the smell of a herb garden, reading and being read to.

As the individual moves through their dementia the activities will move from ones encouraging physical and mental interaction to activities that are much more sensory. Sensory activities are those which play up to the five senses of touch, smell, taste, hearing and sight, finger painting to herb gardens, different textures to stronger tasting foods.

36. Where should people with dementia live?

This is a difficult question to answer because of the emotions present when this decision needs to be taken. We need to plan better and have more options available with clear guidance set down as to when options should be considered based on the individual's needs at that time.

There would appear to be five main options today, these are:

1. Remaining at home.
2. Moving from home to a care setting: either residential, nursing or supported living.
3. Moving to a specialised service caring for people with learning difficulties and dementia from home, care home (either residential, nursing or supported living).
4. Moving into a mainstream nursing home specialising in caring for people with dementia.
5. Transfer from current accommodation to hospital and dying in hospital.

Let's look at one of these options in detail and see the possible issues it raises through a case study.

George is 49 years old and has lived for the last 15 years in a seven-bedded supported living service for people with learning difficulties. The organisation running the home transferred from residential to supported living services four years ago.

George has moderate learning difficulties: his communication skills are good, but he only uses non-verbal communication. However, carers working with George describe him as having capacity to make day-to-day decisions in his life.

Like many services of this type one of their primary aims is to support individuals to maximise their levels of independence and further develop their community presence. George is independent in most areas of his day-to-day life but has little understanding of areas including money and the implications of his health needs. He therefore requires support on a regular basis.

He is assigned support for five hours a day. This support is primarily around finance, medication, doctors or medical appointments, general cooking skills and housekeeping skills.

He travels independently to college where he is on a basic cooking skills course. His medical problems include hypothyroidism, sight and hearing difficulties. He is also susceptible to chest infections.

George has regular visits from his mum and two sisters who take an active interest in his life. They are very happy with his support plan and his development over the last fifteen years. His parents agreed for his move out of the family home as they were planning both for his and their future.

Over the last two months carers have raised concerns over a range of issues including:

- On two occasions he got 'lost' going to college.
- A slight deterioration in self-help skills, e.g. on one occasion he was noted to be wearing the same clothes on two consecutive days, something he had never previously done.
- On one occasion when in town he alarmed the carer supporting him by stepping out into the road without looking. He had never done this before.

Over the next few months more and more incidents of unusual behaviour were recorded, including other service users raising concerns that George doesn't seem himself. During this process George was referred to his GP who carried out the usual barrage of tests. Nothing was found by the tests but as the deterioration continued, he was further referred to the learning disability team. After a range of assessments were completed, dementia was agreed as the most likely cause of the deterioration. This process took six months, which is quite normal and shows thorough assessments have been carried out.

I'd like to look at the impact of this on four different groups:

George

George's future is now mapped out (see answers to Questions 12 and 23). He will move through the stages of dementia over the next three to five years.

His needs will increase in time and his apparent understanding of people and the world around him will diminish. This means over time his needs will increase and he will require more carer time to meet those needs.

This sounds harsh but is the reality of anyone correctly diagnosed with dementia.

Up until now his world was one of change, development and progression. It is now one of change, deterioration and eventually end of life care. But please remember there is lots of quality living still to be had for individuals with dementia. Lots of happy times, smiles and laughs.

Family

Most of the family are slowly coming to terms with the changes in George. They are at times expressing feelings of guilt and anger. One sister is still in denial and is just wanting George to snap out of it and get back to normal; most of the anger expressed is coming from this sister.

The multi-disciplinary team have given the family reading material and website addresses to find out more about dementia. However, we also accept that not all materials are read until the person is ready to accept the reality of the current situation.

They still visit regularly and the care team have set aside time to answer their questions and let them know how George is, and any changes noted. The family are also invited to, and attend, all case reviews held about their son/brother.

It is vitally important to respect the value of working constructively with family. They have so much to offer but for them to be fully involved the team need to keep them informed. It is important to remember to pace our information and recognise the signs of grief in relatives, such as denial and anger. These are normal first reactions for all of us.

There may be some exceptions to this rule, but they are rare, e.g. where the passing on of all the information may cause an already frail elderly relative to become more ill.

Other service users

The six other service users at the home will have had a familiar routine. Having someone in their group with dementia means this routine will change, which can cause confusion.

George, for example, may stop going out to certain set activities in the way he used to. He may forget it is his job to lay the tables for mealtimes. As his needs increase, he may start taking more time from the care team, meaning they get less. This can cause feelings of resentment and jealously.

There are two service users who have autistic-spectrum disorders who may be even more confused as routine is very important for them and deviation may cause confusion and distress. We must involve others who live with the person by giving updates at their level of understanding as to why George is behaving differently from before, within confidentiality boundaries.

Much like working with relatives, we need to be as honest as possible to bring the group along with what is happening.

This will encourage a higher level of communal support for George.

Care/support team

Most people working in a service such as this came into the job with a view to supporting people to learn new skills, promote independence and encourage community involvement.

When one of those individuals develops dementia, the rules and skill set are suddenly changed: the aims for this person are now keeping skills for as long as possible and not teaching new skills.

Where previously family and carers have enjoyed supporting

people to have an increasing community presence, as the person's dementia progresses these opportunities will decrease. Family members and carers will be concentrating on maintaining and promoting quality of life, for as long as possible, in a deteriorating situation.

This is quite a change, which will become more profound as the dementia advances. Consideration needs to be taken if the care team has the skill set to manage this and end of life care when the time comes.

All care teams should put this issue on their agenda now: if one of the service users developed dementia what should they do? Are there new skills they would have to learn? At what stage should they be looking to more specialist services for support or taking over support of the individual?

Many teams I have worked with have not had this discussion before my involvement.

As a result I am often faced with the situation that half the team believe the person should stay where they are until the end of their life and the other half believe strongly that the impact the person is having on other service users means they should move to more specialist services. This is a difficult situation that can damage working relationships within the team.

With more forward thinking, contingency plans can be put in place for an event that is increasingly likely to happen in the foreseeable future.

Organisations who specialise in learning disability, who are currently providing services to people who have Down syndrome over the age of 40, should be planning how this group should be cared for if dementia is diagnosed.

Where a person lives should be dependent on their needs: how their dementia is affecting them balanced against the impact on the other service users and care team or family, if they are living at home. While a person is still aware of where they are and the people within their environment they should stay there for as long as possible. However, the needs of others must be considered equally.

Without forward planning some situations are resolved by others although not necessarily in the person's best, emotional, interest.

For example, if George was living in a seven-bedded service and all bedrooms were upstairs then, if he developed dementia and became unable to manage the stairs, the regulators would require him to be moved. If George's behaviour became less manageable and was having a detrimental effect on the other service users, then again safeguarding teams may insist that his needs could not be met in his current environment.

Both of these examples may result in urgent placement elsewhere which, although they may provide for George's physical needs, might not be in George's best interest.

Some organisations have been forward looking and have developed both nursing homes and specific nursing homes for individuals with learning disability and dementia. Across the country we need more of these types of unit.

The two other options of being transferred to a general nursing home or hospital are my least favoured options. People who have Down syndrome and dementia often have additional needs, especially around communication, that require specialist services and training. Therefore, their care should remain in the learning disability services. In addition, the age of most people in nursing homes and older care wards in hospitals potentially creates additional problems.

This age group are often from a cultural background that believed that people with learning disabilities should be locked away from society in institutions.

This potentially creates an unhealthy mix of service users and under-qualified carers.

If there was better provision within the learning disability sector this would not have to happen.

Politically, the new move towards integrated health and social care needs to look more closely into these issues and produce recommendations that ensure end of life issues for individuals with Down syndrome and dementia are better catered for by a caring society.

The bringing together of organisations in this area and development of an action plan is long overdue. If any such group were to be set up, I would gladly become a member.

Appendix

Useful websites for more information:

1. Downs syndrome Association – www.downs-syndrome.org.uk
2. British Institute of Learning Disabilities – www.bild.org.uk
3. Alzheimer's Society – www.alzheimers.org.uk
4. Alzheimer's Research UK – http://alzheimersresearchuk.org
5. National Down Syndrome Society – www.ndss.org
6. Down's Heart Group – http://dhg.org.uk/information/
7. University of Cambridge Psychiatry Department – http://psychiatry.cam.ac.uk
8. Brief guide: Positive behaviour support for people with behaviours that challenge – www.cqc.org.uk
9. National Library of Medicine – http://www.ncbi.nim.nih.gov
10. Department of Health: Quality outcomes for people with dementia 28th Sept 2010 – https://www.gov.uk/government/publications/quality-outcomes-for-people-with-dementia-building-on-the-work-of-the-national-dementia-strategy
11. Mental Capacity Act 2005 – www.legislation.gov.uk
12. Mental Health Act 2017 – www.legislation.gov.uk
13. Mental Capacity Act 2005 at a glance – https://www.scie.org.uk
14. The Care Act 2014 – www.legislation.gov.uk
15. Guideline 10 – www.nice.org.uk

Afterword

My hope in this book was to answer questions raised in training/development sessions. Have all your questions been answered? If you have any questions that I have not covered please email them to me at bob_dawson@ymail.com. Who knows, but if sufficient questions are raised, I may complete a second book.

I would also love to receive any comments or observations on the book.